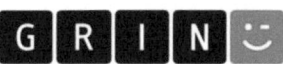

Health and Safety for Airlines. An Example of New Zealand

Damien Hiquet

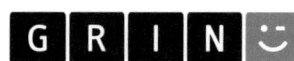

Bibliographic information published by the German National Library:

The German National Library lists this publication in the National Bibliography; detailed bibliographic data are available on the Internet at http://dnb.dnb.de.

ISBN: 9783346543578
This book is also available as an ebook.

Print and binding: Books on Demand GmbH, Norderstedt, Germany
Printed on acid-free paper from responsible sources.

The present work has been carefully prepared. Nevertheless, authors and publishers do not incur liability for the correctness of information, notes, links and advice as well as any printing errors.

GRIN web shop: https://www.grin.com/document/1151088

Airline Occupational Health and Safety Management Practice
Leadership in a New Zealand Context

Damien Hiquet

2021

Table of contents

1. Introduction _____ 3

2. Organisational Governance and Operations _____ 4

2.1 The need to improve _____ 4

2.2 The Benefits _____ 5

3. HSWA 2015 Organisation Roles and Responsibilities _____ 5

3.1 Key terms _____ 5

3.2 Duties of PCBU _____ 6

3.3 Duties of officers, workers, and other persons _____ 6

3.4 Engagement and participation _____ 8

4. Health and Safety Management Systems (HSMS)_____ 8

4.1 Policy and planning _____ 9

4.2 Delivery _____ 9

4.3 Monitoring _____ 11

4.4 Review _____ 12

5. Conclusion _____ 12

References _____ 13

1. Introduction

Hiquet (2021) asserted that "an airline is a complex organisation with multiple management systems, dispersed operations, many technical functions, highly regulated-overlapping State jurisdiction and subject to multiple national regulations " (p. 1) like shown in "figure 1".

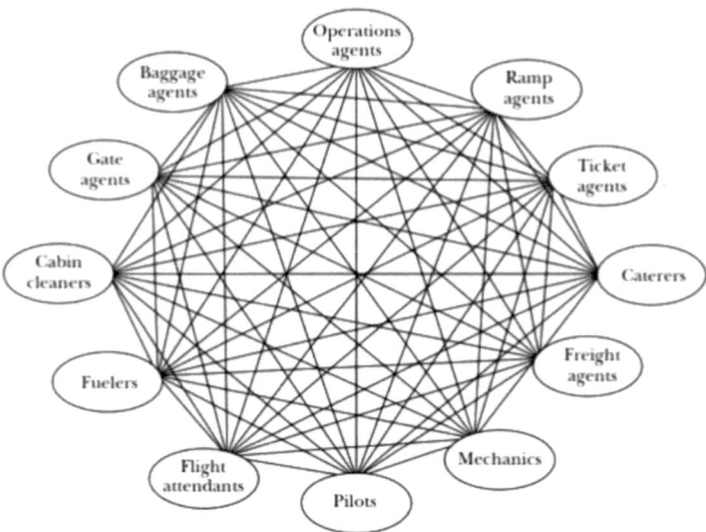

Figure 1: Employee work groups involved in the flight departure process (Bamber et al., 2013, p. 88)

Therefore, senior officers such as the Chief Executive Officer (CEO) and board directors must exercise due diligence on health and safety by having a good understanding of the risk profile of its operations, the key controls in place and a system of providing information on whether these controls are working.

In addition, leaders need to demonstrate to their staff, their suppliers, customers and contractors that they mean it (The Institute of Directors, 2021).

2. Organisational Governance and Operations

2.1 The need to improve

Since 2004, approximately 105 workers are killed annually in Aotearoa from work-related injuries. The broader social and economic impacts of worker fatalities are estimated between fifteen and twenty billions New Zealand Dollars (NZ$) per annum (two to four per cent of gross domestic product).

In New Zealand, work-related fatal injury (WRFI) record has been poor compared with other Organisation for Economic Co-operation and Development (OECD) countries, being twice as high as Australia and four times that of the United Kingdom.

Although, high-profile occupational fatality events such as the Pike River Coal mine tragedy in 2010, have placed Kiwi workplace safety record under public scrutiny (Lilley et al., 2020).

Therefore, the Pike Rover Royal Commission which led to the elaboration of Health and Safety at Work Act 2015 (HSWA) and the creation of WorkSafe New Zealand stated:

"The board and directors are best placed to ensure that the company effectively manages health and safety. They should provide the necessary leadership and are responsible for the major decisions that must influence health and safety: the strategic direction, securing and allocating resources and ensuring the company has appropriate people, systems and equipment" (Institute of Directors in New Zealand, 2013).

As a principle of good governance, the responsibility to have the policy to develop an Occupational Health and Safety Management System (OHSMS) resides in the senior management of the organisation.

2.2 The Benefits

A robust health and safety culture that begins at the board table and spreads throughout the organisation adds significant value.

Indeed, there are benefits linked to having a health and safety culture such as (The Institute of Directors, 2021):

- Enhanced standing among potential workers, customers, suppliers, partners and investors as a result of a good reputation for a commitment to health and safety.
- Workers participating positively in other aspects of the organisation. A good organisational culture spreads wider than health and safety.
- Decreased worker absence and turnover. Engaged workers are more productive workers. For example, it improves productivity as workers feel the management takes OHS seriously by engaging them with their work (Garnicaa & Carsire Barriga, 2018).

For instance, the cost of running an efficient OHSMS is offset by significant savings in insurances premiums and, for organisations part of the Accident Compensation Corporation (ACC) Accredited Employer Programme (AEP), to reduce their levies.

3. HSWA 2015 Organisation Roles and Responsibilities

3.1 Key terms

In section seventeen, the meaning of Person Conducting a business or undertaking (PCBU). For instance, the airline as a legal person. (WorkSafe New Zealand, 2019).

However, the executive team members fulfil the role of an officer as describes in section eighteen and must exercise due diligence to ensure the PCBU meets its health and safety obligations.

In contrast, section nineteen refers to the meaning of worker (e.g., employees/managers, contractors, trainee).

Furthermore, workers have a health and safety duty to take reasonable care to keep themselves and others healthy and safe when carrying out work at the workplace (i.e., section twenty).

For example, an aircraft is a workplace (Parliamentary Office Counsel, 2020).

3.2 Duties of PCBU

In section thirty-six, the organisation has the "primary duty of care" and must ensure, so far as is reasonably practicable (SFAIRP), the health and safety of its workers and any person it influences (e.g., passengers) or directs (e.g., contractors).

If the PCBU manages or controls the workplace (S37) it must ensure, SFAIRP, the workplace, the means of entering and exiting the workplace, and anything else arising from the workplace is without health and safety risks to any person (WorkSafe New Zealand, 2019).

In practice, the primary duty of care is a broad overarching duty that includes, but is not limited to, the organisation having effective practices in place (WorkSafe New Zealand, 2017).

3.3 Duties of officers, workers, and other persons

WorkSafe has charged three individuals under section forty-four of HSWA over the Whakaari/White Island eruption tragedy (ComplyWith, 2020).

Indeed, it imposes a due diligence duty on officers of an organisation, which is a new duty in the HSWA 2015 when it came into force and this is the first WorkSafe prosecution for a breach of it.

Therefore, this section requires the executive team and senior managers, to exercise due diligence to ensure the organisation is complying with all its duties and obligations under the HSWA.

Meanwhile, sections forty-seven to forty-nine describe the offences relating to duties of care and the maximum penalties attached to them.

For instance, a breach can lead to a fine of up to $600,000 and imprisonment for up to five years as stated.

While the facts of any given case will inform what might be construed as "the care, diligence, and skill that a reasonable officer would exercise in the same circumstances", section forty-four also makes some minimum requirements very clear (Parliamentary Office Counsel, 2020) . These include taking reasonable steps to:

- acquire, and keep up-to-date, knowledge of work health and safety matters
- gain an understanding of the nature of the operations of the business or undertaking of the organisation and generally of the associated hazards and risks
- ensure that the organisation has (and uses) appropriate processes
- eliminate or minimise risks to health and safety (and has and uses appropriate resources for this purpose)
- receive and consider information regarding incidents, hazards and risks and respond in a timely way to that information
- comply with any duty or obligation of the organisation under the Act
- verify that these processes are happening and resources are being provided

However, the workers have also a duty to take reasonable care to keep themselves and others healthy and safe when performing work as depicted in section forty-five.

Under section forty-six, other persons in a workplace (e.g., customers) need to take reasonable care that anything they do (or do not do) will not cause other harm.

If they cause someone harm and did not take reasonable care, they can be legally responsible (Taituarā — Local Government Professionals Aotearoa, 2021).

3.4 Engagement and participation

Sections fifty-eight to sixty-one require the PCBU, SFAIRP, to engage with its workers including those carry-out work activities for the organisation, and workers who are or are likely to be, directly affected by a matter relating to the work activities of the PCBU.

Nevertheless, worker engagement and participation practices can be direct or through representation.

For instance, Health and Safety Representatives (HSRs) and Health and Safety Committees (HSCs) are two well-established methods of representation. Workers have rights and PCBU's have obligations towards these representatives and committees.

4. Health and Safety Management Systems (HSMS)

Directors must exercise due diligence to health and safety through their governance role as defined in section forty-four of the HSWA.

Therefore, the role of directors is outlined in four key elements: Policy and planning, delivery, monitoring and review.

As a participant of the ACC AEP, those elements are already a prerequisite for the organisation to join the scheme (Accident Compensation Corporation, 2017) and the process is depicted by Hiquet (2020) as the following (p. 4):

4.1 Policy and planning

In the first principle of AS/NZS 4804:2001, the commitment of the senior management to the goal of the OHSMS must be manifested in the company policy and is continually reiterated by the things that management pay attention to and measure.

Furthermore, that health and safety culture must reflect in the organisation policy (Safety Institute of Australia, 2012).

4.2 Delivery

For aviation operations, a Safety Management System (SMS) provides a systematic approach for reducing risks to an acceptable level by reducing their probability and/ or consequence.

Therefore, the SMS is designed to be a dynamic foundation that goes beyond compliance to continually improve safety performance by enhancing proactive management of change, operational efficiencies and employee engagement.

However, airlines have multiple management systems supported by different departments.

In 2006, the International Civil Aviation Organisation (ICAO) published the Safety Management Manual (SMM) which required airlines to implement an SMS through their national bodies (i.e., New Zealand Civil Aviation Authority) and stated that "Aviation organization should be encouraged to integrate their quality, safety, security, occupational health and safety, and environmental management systems" (ICAO, 2008).

Consequently, the company has adopted an Integrated Airline Safety Management System (IASMS) which acts as a dashboard by providing measurable operational safety performance indicators (Royal NLR, n.d.) and key health and safety lead indicators to be reviewed weekly by the executive team (Safe+, 2017).

Within this model, the HSMS sits under the General Manager of People Safety and Aviation Medicine while the IASMS focuses more on operational safety and consequently is under the helm of the Chief Operational Integrity and Safety Officer.

In the aviation context, the organisation must comply with operations covered by an aviation certificate (e.g., ground and flight operations, aircraft maintenance) and the Health and Safety at Work Act 2015 (HSWA) for activities outside the scrutiny of the CAA.

Nevertheless, these safety systems are complementary.

Meanwhile, the executive team has developed a Health, Safety, Environment and Wellbeing Management System (HSEW) which provide the organisation with a dynamic foundation focused on holistic management from the bottom-up (i.e., CEO) to managing people safety where they are all equally accountable ("Figure 2").

Due to quality issues this image was removed by the editorial staff.

Figure 2: Components of the HSEW management system

The components make up a crucial part of the HSEW management system and all work together and have an inter-related influence on the other components within the system.

While the system framework is based on the three pillars (risk, relationships and resources), it is reviewed annually (in line with the corporate strategic planning cycle) and enhanced on a regular cycle of three years.

Finally, the framework is developed in collaboration with the workforce (i.e, employees and unions), learnings from past years and integrated within corporate governance and aligned to achieve organisational strategy.

As the operating components are supported by a process platform to ensure only what matters to the employee is monitored (Business Leaders Health & Safety Forum, 2019).

4.3 Monitoring

With the HSWA 2015, the Crown shifts the focus from monitoring and recording health and safety incidents to proactively identifying and managing risks so workers are safe and healthy (Worksafe, 2017).

For instance, the organisation promotes a Just Culture approach by encouraging reporting (e.g., incidents, hazards) investigation, sharing, and implementation of learnings from the event which is guided by the event management model:
1. Emergency response
2. Initial actions
3. Investigation
4. Corrective and preventative actions (i.e., continuous improvement)

Nevertheless, events are categorised to provide analysis and decision making (e.g., Operational Safety Request (OSR), hazard).

4.4 Review

The PCBU adheres to AS/NZ4804:2001 and its fifth principle states the organisation should regularly review and continually improve its HSMS, to improve its health and safety performance for the HSMS to mature at the same pace as the organisation and to be integrated into all business decisions based on measurable data.

Therefore, it is an important component of corporate governance to ensure that the HSMS meet the requirements of the organisation policy.

5. Conclusion

The organisation has capitalised on the elaboration of an efficient HSMS that integrates international standards and obey health and safety national regulations which fence the power and responsibility of the executive team.

For instance, the pre-requisite of internal audits from the AEP scheme gives the executives an overview of what happens inside the company and to take corrective and preventive actions and the HSWA reminds them of the penalties they could face.

Besides, psychological safety needs to be promoted amongst the workforce and participation encouraged.

However, leaders have to lead by example and the culture of health and safety needs to be driven from the top down.

To conclude, these are the three questions ending all messages of the CEO of Air New Zealand to its staff: "Is it safe to start work? How do you know?What if you are wrong? Safe On-Time Performance (OTP) only counts if it is achieved safely."

.

References

Accident Compensation Corporation. (2017). *Accredited Employers Programme.* ACC. https://www.acc.co.nz/assets/business/acc440-aep-audit.pdf

Bamber, Greg J., et al. *Up in the Air : How Airlines Can Improve Performance by Engaging Their Employees,* Cornell University Press, 2011. ProQuest Ebook Central, https://ebookcentral.proquest.com/lib/sitlibrary-ebooks/detail.action? docID=3137995.

Business Leaders Health & Safety Forum. (2019, May). *Monitoring what matters. Business Leaders' Health & Safety Forum* – Bringing leaders together with a common vision for ZeroHarm Workplaces. https://www.zeroharm.org.nz/assets/ docs/our-work/monitoring/Monitoring-What-Matters-May2019.pdf

Hiquet, D. (2021). *MGT 226 Occupational Health and Occupational Safety Training Strategies and Evaluation. Assignment One* [Unpublished manuscript]. Southern Institute of Technology.

ICAO. (2008, October 2). Introduction to SMS. https://www.icao.int/safety/afiplan/ Documents/Safety%20Management/2008/SMS%20Workshop/Modules/ ICAO%20SMS%20Module%20N°%207%20 %20Introduction%20to%20SMS%202008-11%20(E).pdf

International Labour Office. *Guidelines on Occupational Safety and Health Management Systems : ILO-OSH 2001,* International Labour Office, 2001. ProQuest Ebook Central, http://ebookcentral.proquest.com/lib/sitlibrary-ebooks/detail.action? docID=359379.

Lilley, R., Maclennanh, B., McNoe, B. M., Davie, G., Horsburgh, S., & Driscoll, T. (2020, March 24). *Decade of fatal injuries in workers in New Zealand: insights from a*

Damien Hiquet

comprehensive national observational study. Injury Prevention | A BMJ journal on
the burden of injury.
https://injuryprevention.bmj.com/content/injuryprev/27/2/124.full.pdf

Parliamentary Office Counsel. (2020). *Health and Safety at Work Act 2015 no 70 (as at 01*
December 2020), Public Act contents – New Zealand legislation (70).
https://www.legislation.govt.nz/act/public/2015/0070/latest/
DLM5976660.html#DLM5976848

Royal NLR. (n.d.). *Safety performance indicators.* https://www.nlr.org/capabilities/safety-
performance-indicators/

Safe+. (2017). *Lead indicators.Examples across industry sectors.* WorkSafe. https://
worksafe.govt.nz/dmsdocument/3350-lead-indicators

Safety Institute of Australia. (2012, April). Systems. The OHS Body of Knowledge. https://
www.ohsbok.org.au/wp-content/uploads/2013/12/11-Systems.pdf

Taituarā — Local Government Professionals Aotearoa. (2021). *Module one, part E -*
Duties and rights of workers and other persons. Welcome to the
LGSectorGoodToolkit® » Taituarā. https://www.solgm.co.nz/health-and-safety-at-
work/module-one-part-e-duties-and-rights-of-workers-and-other-persons/

The Institute of Directors in New Zealand. (2013, May). *Good governance practices*
guideline for managing health and safety risks. Business Leaders' Health & Safety
Forum – Bringing leaders together with a common vision for ZeroHarm
Workplaces. https://www.zeroharm.org.nz/assets/docs/news-releases/Directors-
Guidlines-on- Health- and-Safety.pdf

The Institute of Directors. (2021, May 26). *Health and safety governance guide | IoD NZ.*
https://www.iod.org.nz/resources-and-insights/guides-and-resources/health-and-
safety-governance-guide/#

Damien Hiquet

WorkSafe New Zealand. (2017, September 4). *Health and Safety at Work Act 2015.* ———
WorkSafe. https://www.worksafe.govt.nz/laws-and-regulations/acts/hswa/

WorkSafe New Zealand. (2017, October 24). *What is the primary duty of care?* WorkSafe.
    https://www.worksafe.govt.nz/managing-health-and-safety/getting-started/
    understanding-the-law/primary-duty-of-care/what-is-the-primary-duty-of-care/

WorkSafe New Zealand. (2019, July 18). *Introduction to the Health and Safety at Work Act
    2015 – special guide.* WorkSafe. https://www.worksafe.govt.nz/managing-health-
    and-safety/getting-started/introduction-hswa-special-guide/

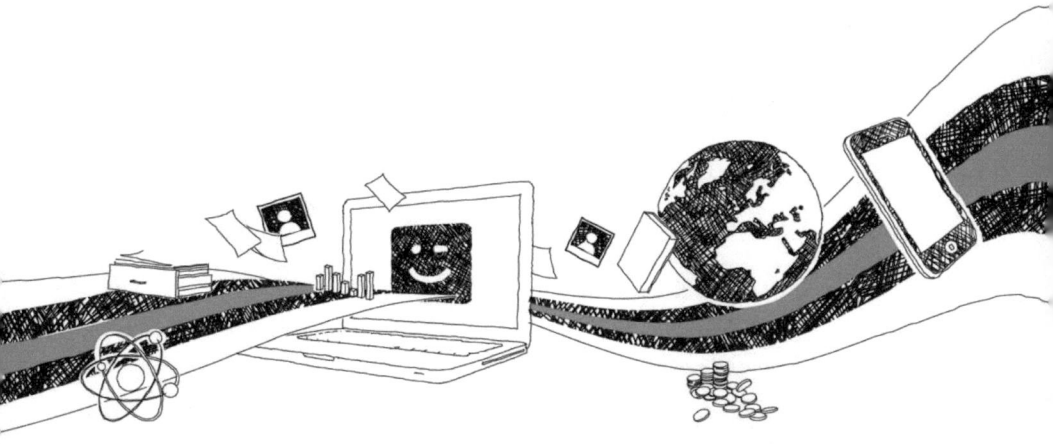
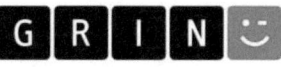